YOUR KNOWLEDGE HAS VALUE

Mukasa Aziz Hawards

Foundations of Professional Writing in Public Health

Concepts in Professional Writing

GRIN Verlag

Bibliografische Information der Deutschen Nationalbibliothek:

Die Deutsche Bibliothek verzeichnet diese Publikation in der Deutschen National-
bibliografie; detaillierte bibliografische Daten sind im Internet über http://dnb.d-
nb.de/ abrufbar.

Imprint:

Copyright © 2013 GRIN Verlag GmbH
Druck und Bindung: Books on Demand GmbH, Norderstedt Germany
ISBN: 978-3-656-54327-5

This book at GRIN:

http://www.grin.com/en/e-book/264198/foundations-of-professional-writing-in-
public-health

GRIN - Your knowledge has value

Der GRIN Verlag publiziert seit 1998 wissenschaftliche Arbeiten von Studenten, Hochschullehrern und anderen Akademikern als eBook und gedrucktes Buch. Die Verlagswebsite www.grin.com ist die ideale Plattform zur Veröffentlichung von Hausarbeiten, Abschlussarbeiten, wissenschaftlichen Aufsätzen, Dissertationen und Fachbüchern.

Visit us on the internet:

http://www.grin.com/

http://www.facebook.com/grincom

http://www.twitter.com/grin_com

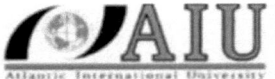

STUDENT NAME: **MUKASA AZIZ**

COURSE NAME: Foundations of Professional Writing in Public Health

Essay Title:

"Developing the Intellectual, scientific Writing Skills"

ATLANTIC INTERNATIONAL UNIVERSITY

October 2013

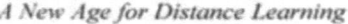
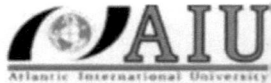

Atlantic International University
A New Age for Distance Learning

Table of Contents

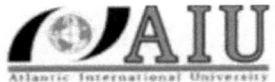
Course Description

This course provides the learner with an opportunity to know and learn about all aspects of writing techniques for use in graduate school as well as in the workplace. The course includes common grammar and spelling errors, writing styles, the ethics of authorship, reference and citation systems, and guidance for scientific communication.

Course Objectives

By the end of this course in scientific professional writing, it's my intention to have obtained the following competences;

1. Locate and evaluate the information from a variety of peer-reviewed publications.
2. Write abstracts and short public health briefs.
3. Learn a variety of ways to present public health issues.
4. Explore public health issues that may or may not be of interest to your field of study, i.e. financial, ethical, social, behavioral, medical and environmental topics.
5. Understand how to work in small discussion groups to maximize product development while minimizing time.

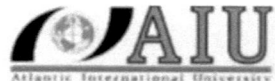
1.0   Introduction

Communication is a process of interacting involving the sharing and transfer of information amongst individuals that could be in proximity or at distant locations. The fact acknowledging the interactive nature of human beings also further affirms that the aspect of communication is inbuilt and not an acquired one at any time in life. However, being inborn does not mean that it remains fixed at a certain point but rather due to various dynamics in life communication undergoes development from one stage and it is this loyal concept that has allowed communication to modify into the sophiscated models observed in today's civilization.

History has it that the ancient medieval world though currently considered to be old fashioned and somewhat primitive lifestyle yet evidence from fossils, astrology, has provided millions of ancient origin manuscripts containing written records in form of symbols, insignias, signs, and drawn compositions relating to communication amongst different parties. In this consideration the modern person of today's world of civilization will boastfully disregard the ancient work and their contribution towards our current literature only if he fails to realize that writing has only developed into the current standards but was initially started by the human predecessors of the ancient generations.

To eliminate this form of useless anonymity from our beliefs we should consider for instance the ancient civilization of Egypt where currently the astrologic discoveries have consequently discovered the writings on the walls and the Chinese calligraphy where both of these are core cornerstones in the development of art and active communication through written form and material. (American Medical Association Manual of Style, 1998)

Writing is basically a skill involving the scribing marks, symbols, drawings and diagrams on any material where it can be realized, interpreted and used for some future reference by different parties. Writing can be used for various purposes of expression, interaction, and communication while using the suitable parameters (symbols, marks, signs, diagrams, drawings) that hold basic meaning of that very time and can be used to transfer knowledge and information to the next generation.

The study of the basic concepts in writing involves or constitutes understanding the underlying key guidelines mapping the idea of writing in the professional practice that can eminently be used to result into effective and remarkable significance in the public health paradigm. In addition, this course further explores the issue of knowledge transfer, rationale of the writing and knowledge transfer process or paradigm, concepts of the modern APA style of scientific writing, administrative presentation of written information, the aspects of authenticity, privacy and intellectual property as recommended by the international standards.

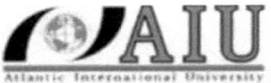
Henceforth, the cardinal importance of this study scope is to ensure discretion and promote intellectual development or confidence for the source party in relation to the international recommended standards of professional and scientific writing norms.

2.0 Chapter One
Key Aspects of Communication in the Public Health Paradigm

2.1 The Rationale of Communication in Public Health
The public health sector faces a great challenge which could possibly be more precarious than the haunted epidemics and this is the poor developments in communication patterns and norms around the globe. The western world has the resources onto which it can stand to boast over their counterparts in the poor states where literature and civilization are still in their primary stages and raw status. At this point, it should be noted that communication undergoes development and the lesser the stage the more inefficient it is in solving public affairs.

Communication is a cardinal aspect in the inter-relationships amongst individuals as it serves a great role in improving transparency which is a precursor for stewardship and trust. Though differences might arise in the due process of interacting parties yet these will result into negligible effects towards the relationship of the two communicating parties. For in case of improper bilateral relations between parties, the cause of their difference can be attributed to miscommunications and misconceptions that could be possibly existing at both sides. However, if the trusting party consider its counterpart to be 'playing by the rules' then there will be a high tendency of openness or professional transparency as the trustee considers his information safe and well protected by the preserved guidelines. Further still, it can still be postulated that in case of contention propaganda can be adopted in its compatible format of either white, grey or black propaganda if in case it is the only tool to cause stability equilibrium.

Effective and guided communication ensures the security of accountability or responsiveness of the trusted party towards the public. Most especially if the written format of communication is taken under serious considerations it is actualized that it contains a great deal of consistence and seigniorial renderings to individuals of reference in an organisation and these will take great care in order to eliminate any possibility of faulting so that their accountability and position is not compromised (Colomb, & Williams, 1985).

The prescriptions offered by the pharmacist to the patient for example if the patient responds negatively to an extent of fatal results then it will be the written prescriptions that will redeem the medic or indict his person as a 'quack'. The forensics certainly analyse the cause of death and the postmortem results will finalize with ingestion of the chemical compound that certainly could be the cause of death. However, at all these levels nowhere does the medic make part of the

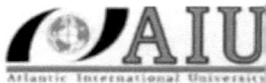
equation not until the last given prescriptions indicate wrong directives and hence at this point the medic is made accountable for the inaccuracy (American Medical Association Manual of Style, 1998).

Further still, it is the role of communication to promote easiness and simplicity in causing public awareness of the health threatening developments and breakouts. In so many cases the epidemiology reports have been published at particular significant time intervals through which the public health sector demonstrates the prevalence of health and advocates for strategic changes in communities aimed at promoting preventive health care.

Another important reason to support the significant role played by communication in promoting health is the channeling of policy development through the different stakeholders for consultation, supplementation and implementation. Policy development is a very important item in the public health sector as it contains the elements that are to construct an effective task force ad formulate an achievable strategy though all these stages require equivocal avenues and involvement of the community and the technocrats from the different health sectors who also constitutes the common stakeholders. The eminent role that communication will predominantly play in this process is to stage up all the ambitious groups into this stake and help in the alignment of the proposed strategies until all the parties reach a fundamental agreement.

2.2 Why Written Communication?

A lot of written material has been saturated all the market halls and media centers arranged in form of organizational bulletins, newspapers, magazines, book publications and other format of written editorial material displaying and containing information on awareness in health education and health or even on matters of social concern while others are for knowledge acquisition and transfer. The reason for querying the position of writing in the public health paradigm mainly rotates its resulting roles and key advantages as compared to other forms communication exchange such as the sign and oral modes of communication (Colomb, & Williams, 1985) .

The reason of this argument in this case needs not to be mistaken as only aimed at pointing out how excellent and resourceful can written formats of communication are in public health but more surprisingly it functions to examine or assess it value and fundamental importance. This therefore means that the notion of comparison has to be borrowed and used to outline the differences, weaknesses, and avenues of strength together with the other forms of communication. For better comprehension of the comparative trends between written, oral and sign communication, a differential table can be asserted and parameters of consideration are selected at a random process from those considered to be of great significance in the communication process.

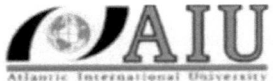
The basic modes of communication to be compared are written, oral or spoken and sign. The basic parameters of comparison within these modes can base on some of those factors discussed earlier as causers for the need to use written communication other than the other forms. Some of these factors include;

1. Target accuracy
2. Compatibility
3. Cost effectiveness
4. Circulation speed and patterns
5. Coverage extent
6. Durability
7. Convenience

Table 1: Showing Comparisons between Written Information and Oral with Sign Formats Of Communication

Assessment parameter	Modes of information transfer		
	Oral method	Written format	Sign language
1. Target accuracy	It effectively strikes the intended groups of individuals though eliminates the deaf	Only the literate and elite groups are reached regardless of the intended group	It is effective in reaching the intended groups of minorities in the community
2. Coverage	It can cover a relatively large area though reduces with increase in regions	Coverage depends on the development in the infrastructure	Very limited
3. Durability	Its degree of consistency reduces with time	It is consistent in nature	Its consistency is extremely unreliable
4. Cost effectiveness	Requires expenses of audio media	Writing material is relatively cheaper	Require a visual transmission media
5. Convenience	Eliminates the aspect of privacy	It strengthens privacy	It is a form of coded language requiring special skills

The table characteristics are derived not on general settings of the public after all these modes can be carried out using electronic or digital media i.e. radio or audio messages, writing material and visual display systems and through television or video transmissions. However, we are trying to compare while looking at these factors under a common organizational setting within

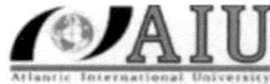
the demarcated enclosures or boundaries since it will present a challenge in determining the far-reaching effects of each mode at an open public setting.

All these parameters under consideration are very wide and their exposition requires visiting different avenues of the current human society for instance, technology developments if considered they can place all these modes of communication on the level of speed, coverage, saturation and convenience and yet at the same time all of them are victims of piracy or ethical violations. (Colomb, & Williams, 1985)

➤ *Development of the communication work plan*

Written communication in the public health setting plays a role of designing a communication framework that can be used to raise awareness, transfer and present knowledge to the designated public where critical insurgences arises. The public health professional encounters challenges of pandemic outbreaks, non-communicable disease prevalence and detrimental health disparities which conceptually alter the stability of the normal work plan. However, with a precise written communication framework in place preventive measures can easily be advocated towards the public which through the campaign easily and quickly adapts descriptive message and implement it instantly. In other words, written communication which also has a feature of consistence will tentatively allow a uniform grasping of the information by the different parties as long as the written remarks are easily perceptible and interpretable by the majority.

➤ *Structuring the general organizational work schedules*

In the intellectual setting, the work schedules and activity or work plans are best displayed to the public and the staff in written format which conceptually holds a visual aspect and sight attention. Individuals in proximity due to less strain required to view the displayed information in the close range further enlarge the importance of written information transfer. For what is private will possibly not be pined for public notice or rather given the information which might raise public discomfort, the predicaments resulting from the circulation of such can only be averted while using the writing norms which accurately upholds the aspect of secrecy as paramount (Gopen, 1990).

2.3 What is writing?

Typically, all forms of writing have a fundamental feature of being visual marks or representations on a surface material e.g. tablet of wood paper. However, this sort of description can be considered to be selective as it excludes the braille modes of writing used for the blind which are tactile in nature other forms of visual representations hence more citation can considerably be asserted that later includes these forms of writing have nothing to do with mere visual marks. The fundamental node that protrudes the essence of writing is that writing consists of a conventional principle in which it carries meaning to a particular extent and this meaning

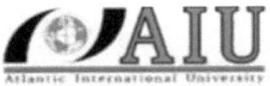
can easily be interpreted by a certain group of individuals. Further still, it should also be noted that visual representations and marks like those produced by the unlearned infant playing with crayons while producing zigzag and revolving threads of lines on a white paper.

However, this kind of presentation holds in itself the aspect of being visual marks on a surface it does not necessarily qualify to a writing simply it holds no meaning and hence nonconventional or lacks a classification group under which it would be interpreted. Nevertheless, this may not still imply that all conventional representations are literally writing in nature take for instance a drawing representation of the sky or the geographical topography of the distant landscape.

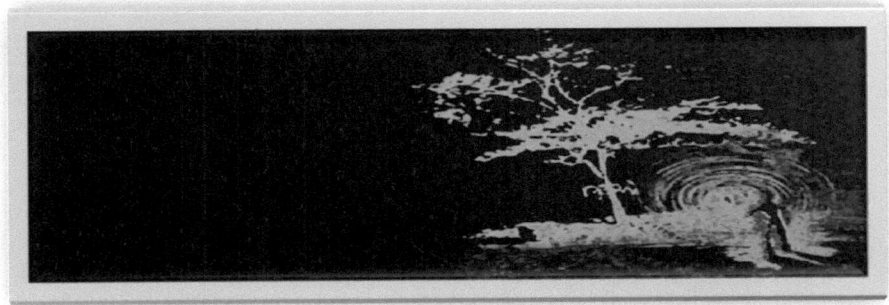

Figure 1: showing a field tunnel perspective in an artistic representation

The ideal reason onto which considerations can be made to eliminate the above representation from the norm of writing is the fact writing always conveys general meaning perhaps to a considerable extent or degree depending on the event time during which that particular mosaic form is adapted.

Further still the aspect of language composition is another factor or underlying feature onto which writing should be considered and this if technically considered further outweighs the visual marks that have some conventional representation. Take for instance the visual mark representing a crossing road section containing infant images running across the sideways.

Figure 2: showing terminal road crossing section sign on the highway for pedestrians

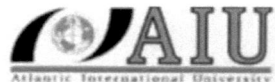
These are visual images built up in a composition format used to represent some event but still this does not qualify the representation to be writing due to the essence of language. In a brief summation, writing has the following characteristics;

❖ Writing consists of visual marks on any given material where they can be recognised regardless of time
❖ Writing in its nature is always read out either loudly or quietly by sub vocalization
❖ The written marks must be representing something understandable and relevant to interpretation
❖ Any form of writing must be attached to a certain language system adapted by a particular community

3.0   Chapter Two
Fundamental concepts in writing

3.1 The History of Writing

The origin and evolution of writing was triggered off by man himself in the medieval periods of the early predecessors, though this theory does not guarantee the assertion that writing started instantly as man had started existing. However, as conceptualized earlier that writing is a skill that undergoes development, then it is agreeable that the invent of writing evolved from dynamic revolutions of the human civilization. During these civilization different inventions were sown among which was the art of drawing as a form of written communication and this has given birth to the actual writing that has been embraced by today's generation.

However, there is extremely shocking evidence that shows a transition which happened in the field of writing over the ancient periods that saw material change, mark development, symbolic representations, notational development and the emergence of alphabets though all these dynamic changes emerged not from a single region and certainly also from across vast spaces of periods.

The historian have been able to identify and establish certainly a numerous number of ancient civilization that show different forms of writing and these have little or completely nothing in common (Gopen, 1990). These have further been depended on to assert that have a remarkable claim on the invent of writing in the different regions of the world and these can be analyzed in the following lines;

(a) The ancient Mesopotamian region from where evolved the **Sumerian writing** in the years around 3200BC. This is considered to be the most ancient and certainly to have given birth to the Egyptian writing system after all they both share the place of origin which could provide

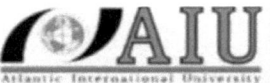
the remains of the ancestral legends and these used for reference by the next generation to develop something new and compatible to their lifestyles. The Sumerian writing system however, concentrated in the Babylonian empire (modern day Iraq) as initially employed by the royal scribes in the temples.

It was a writing system that required special training for a period of time during which the administrative scribes learnt to present words correctly which also further proves that by this time the standardization of pictorial sign had technically emerged and was in usage.

The Sumerian system of writing consisted of about 1000 different signs in which case each one of these signs could even be applied to represent more than one word and this was possibly supported by the help of the rebus principle.

The inscriptions of the Sumerian writing were formerly presented on clay tablets by shaped moldings hence the classical name *cuneiform* that comes from the Latin word *cuneus* for clay.

Sumerian later developed a language but all these were later deformed as they became more complex and hence replaced by the Akkadian word system. However, Sumerian lasted for a prolonged period of about 3000 years with the most recent text dating from 74AD and it supported the language writing in Babylonian, Assyrian, indo- European languages (Hittite, Persian, Elamite and Hurrian).

However, the time systems of both the Egyptian and the Sumerian writings is a great area of intellectual discount because some history like that of the Bible asserts that the Egyptian civilization existed before the Babylonian empire hence it seems to be the origin and not the Babylonian which emerged a thousand years later. Nevertheless the characteristics of these two writing systems have great differences which eliminates the idea that perhaps they could have co-existed in the same time hence came after the other.

Figure 3: showing the clay tablets of the Sumerian language from ancient Babylon

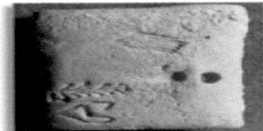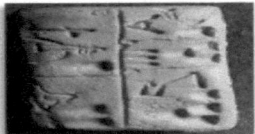

Source: from the Martin Schøyen collection in Norway

(b) The yellow river region **Chinese writing** that emerged before 1200BC and has lasted till today's civilization and the precursor of the artistic calligraphic style.

The Chinese writing have been ascribed as logographic in nature and one of the still existing prototypes made up with a variety of characters. It can be considered that almost all the characters in the Chinese language represent a monosyllabic morpheme i.e. a single sign or character 朩 pronounced as *mu'* with the meaning of 'wood' though this is rarely used as a free word. 朩

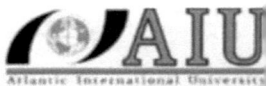
But it should noted that not all the characters in the Chinese language represent morphemes but just some are exist as loanwords in which cases a single character is combined with other notations on the left or right of which none of these represents a morpheme of its own.

Another principle characteristic of the Chinese writing is that a single character represents a singular syllable as it exists in a certain phrase or in other words (polysyllabic morpheme), it has its own independent pronunciation and sound regardless of the surrounding characters.

(c) The Mesoamerican writing which existed in Guatemala and in the southern Mexico briefly after 500BC

Little details have been presented as evidence to ascertain the characteristics of this writing system and worst still its life span or existence is sometimes exaggerated and supported by some religious denominations such as the Moronians.

3.2 The Birth of Writing in Egypt

The Egyptian writing share a lot of originality with the Sumerian type where both have 3000BC as their common time setting but still fundamentally different in style and representation. The fundamental characteristic of the Egyptian ancient writing is that it was so much pictorial and little changes happened to this trend even within the next 3500years of its existence. However, in most cases these signs used represented sounds rather than words hence quietly undecipherable as compared to other forms of writing from the ancient times for example the Sumerian, which is the opposite. The characteristic parameters that are contained in the ancient Egyptian writing system constituted the following aspects;

(i)   The logographic aspect in which case a sign was used to represent or mean an object, word or sound such as @ for r' 'sun' and * for s*b*' 'star'.

(ii)   Consonantal where by a given sign represents a singular or multiple consonants e.g ◖

   For n*b* and   ✗ for s*b*

(iii)   Determinative in which case a figure of a flat lying human indicating the aspect of death. The figure below is of an ancient Egyptian tablet showing a composition of determinative pictorial signs that could have been arranged to narrate an instruction, poem, story or any form of composition to someone.

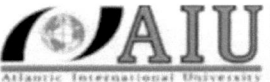
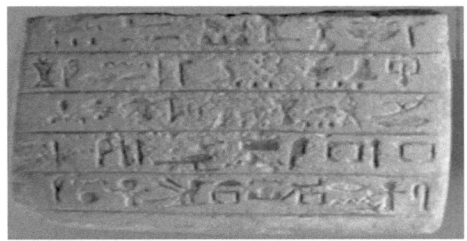

Figure 4: Showing an ancient Egyptian tablet with a composition of numerous signs (extracted from the online encyclopedia)

The Egyptian writing as you navigate through its features it is discovered that vowels were never catered for or excluded which shows some sort of limitations since words could only be constructed from flat consonants hence an idea that these consonants might have some of their origin from this civilization such as in Hebrew, Arabic, and Phoenician.

3.3 The origin of the alphabets in Phoenicia and Greece
The skill of phonographic initially existed with the former Sumerian and the Egyptian civilization though during these periods it was still underscored in usage but developed with time and knowledge. However, the most important developments in the phonographic trends of written communication were most developed in the Phoenician times of the 2nd millennium BC which also produced the early Phoenician alphabet system.

The Phoenician alphabet system was composed of 22 consonants which were the principle cornerstones for the phonographic codes i.e. the consonants represented a particular sound and it had a specific and identifying name. these consonants were independent and it is evident indicated that the current Latin alphabets must have been derived from the Phoenician systems indirectly. Nevertheless, where the Phoenician obtained their alphabet system is still a mystery though historical analysis and together with the technological development of crystal methods relates this origin to the Egyptian roots.

The Greeks studied the Phoenician system of writing from which they introduced a little different alphabet system that had the vowels included hence a fundamental feature that isolated it from the consonantal filled Phoenician method. These went further to combine the vowels with the consonants to formulate word joints, introduction of new consonants, diacritic sign formations in order to express accent and pronunciations and finally this evolution and development indicated the emergence of a new perfect phonemic system of writing and the first of its kind in history (Eva Von Dassow, n.d.).

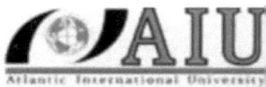

Later on the standard alignment of writing from left to right emerged in the 5th century BC, which replaced the right to left alignment formerly used by the Phoenicians.

Though it is not yet affirmatively asserted that the vowel development emerged from the Macedonian civilization and conquest (Greek Empire) there is strong evidence that connects the ancient writing system in the Greek remains to the likeness of some vowels though this is not final proof of the theory. Some cultures however, even to up to date are still maintaining the principle dominance of the consonants over the vowels which has actually been adapted as the standard whereas others have excluded the vowels such as the Hebrew writing system as shown in the pure consonant characters below.

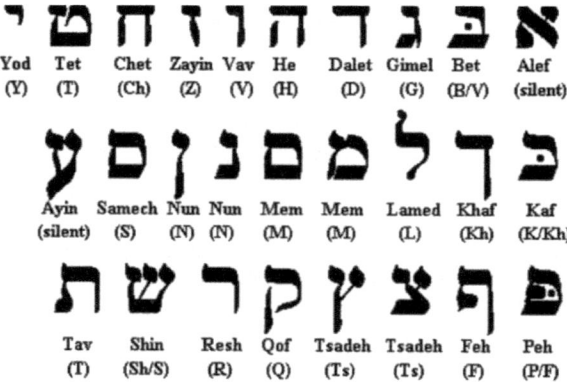

The Hebrew pure consonant writing system (*Adopted from the Martin Schøyen collection in Norway*)

3.4 The Elements of Writing

For standard settings in the writing arenas it has been conceptualized by linguists that certain rules should be followed while in setting up groups of writing patterns. These rules act as the underlying principles onto which the ancient forms of writings can be classified for better analysis and study purposes. The writing system therefore, can be described as the a set of rules or even principles denoted to a given signs written relating to a certain linguistic criteria which can either a sound or any other form of meaning.

Technically it has been postulated that the writing systems all over the various generations can be differentiated according to either the script used or the underlying rules. In addition it can even be possible that the two differing types of writings have none in common either in script or

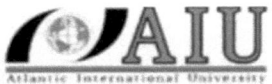
in the underlying principles. The script can be described as the set of the physical written signs relating to a particular meaning or sound in a given language.

Take for instance the comparison between the Korean and the Indian writing systems in this case which show resemblance in a certain pattern. Under critical scrutiny, it can be idealized that the Korean writing system derives all its underlying principles from the Indian trend though the scripts or characters used in Korean are extremely different. In this case, the Korean writing has scripts, which share pronunciation, syllable combination and sounds like the Indian types but the shape of these characters are totally different. On the other hand, the Greek and the Chinese set of writing share none of the script or underlying principles. In addition to scripts and underlying principles the elements of writing are detailed below;

1. Writing system for example the digraphia and the mixed writing system
2. Scripts which are the set of written signs carrying linguistic meaning
3. Case sensitive where the upper case is used to capitalize the word or introduce a new sentence or proper names as used in the Greek alphabets
4. Character styles for example plain, cursive, **bold,** underlined, etc. such renderings can be used to indicate emphasis or any other aspect of communication
5. Punctuation marks for instance; <?>, <!>, <.>,<,>, etc. they are used in grammatical assembling of sentences to aid in parsing, clauses, mark between declarative and interrogative sentences, to demarcate emotional aspects etc.
6. Direction of the characters; This element is flexible depending on the region and culture aspect. However, the most common directions of writing are;
    i.   Left to right lines while descending from top to bottom
    ii.   Right to left lines descending from the top to the bottom
    iii. Top to bottom lines running from right to left

The standard and globally recommended alignment of lines in the intellectual writing has been the left-right lines running from the top to the bottom.

3.5 Types of Writing
The development of linguistics and the writing paradigm in the various professional arenas provides most of the apparent basis to establish the distinction in writing. However, the ancient legendary scribes and history tellers intended not to create difference between each other's work there are considerable "signatures" in their written content that provides room for disagreement and hence showing no point of consortium among these ancient written works.

The modern studies have enabled the discovery of these differences and it has been conceptualized that the writing systems show distinctions on parameters of morphemes,

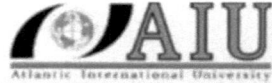
syllables, phonemes and the meaning of conventional relationships. The main types of writing are;

- ❖ **Logographic** writing system: - this type of writing system is currently demonstrated in Chinese literature. Logographic writing involves the use of a single unit of the script such as a sign to represent a particular meaning in which could either be a word or a morpheme.
  As explained earlier that in the Chinese writing system or pattern each character has a morphemic identity even when there has been a combination of another character.

- ❖ **Phonographic** writing system: - This type of writing system dominates the modern used approach universally. In phonologic writing each sign or script is just phonetic in nature and therefore carries no significant conventional meaning. Being phonetic in nature implies that a unit sign is possibly is mere sound in the word pronunciation that can certainly be used to separate it from another word having the same "features."

However, phonologic writing can further be differentiated into syllabic or phonemic in nature in which case the unit sign is a mere syllable or a phoneme. In the syllabic writing style therefore, a single sign represents the sound of a unit vowel just like in the Japanese language yet in phonemic style that is followed in the Latin alphabet and our common English language.

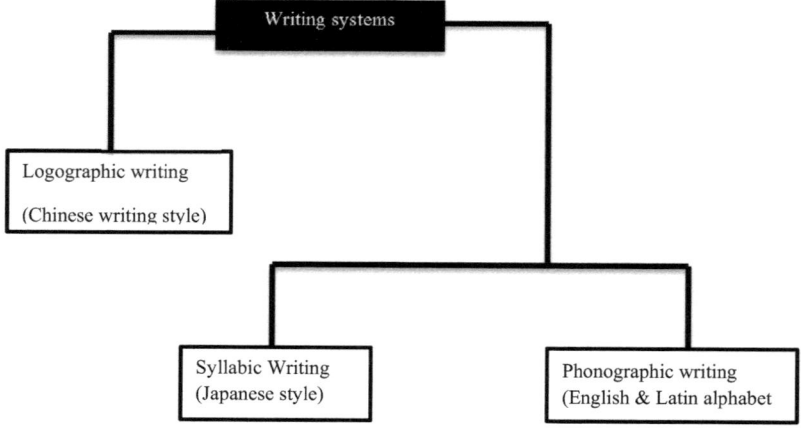

Figure 5: flow chart showing the examples and types of writing systems

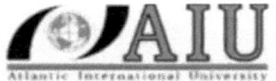
4.0   **Chapter Three**

Concepts in Professional Writing and Development of Intellectual Skills

4.1 Intellectual Considerations

The presentation of the information in written form is in most cases a result of final analysis that has been fully edited and therefore is considerably applicable for reference and reproof as need may call. Due to this fact in the intellectual development paradigm, it is vital to concentrate on the formatting skills that can enable a professional practitioner to produce a remarkably dependable and effective written information that is to be used by the public for different purposes.

There is a degree of preciseness that should be represented in the written work either electronic, digital or paper presentation and this can be attained after a critical considerations of factors before embarking on the writing process. Some of the most critical factors include the following;

1. Audience

At so many times we encounter readings that offsets our attention or arouse us to extents we dint imagine from the start point. It is very important to identify the type of audience that is targeted by the written work and what their encounter will face. At times we are compelled assume that the our audience are well acquainted with the knowledge and acronyms of the subject and hence tempted to neglect background information and excessive usage of acronyms that might certainly be unknown to the reader (Blackwell, & Martin, 2011).

Examples for analyzing the audience should include; the irrelevance or awareness towards the topic and knowledge of the acronyms. These considerations help in discussing or explain the necessary parts to the topic to the audience and at the same time saves the time would have wasted in explaining the commonly-known issues and acronyms to the audience.

2. Alignment standards

Most of the common organizations have standard and recommended structure of documentation followed while addressing various occasions in the company process and dynamics and these sometimes are kept in form of templates for future reference. It is unadvisable for any official document on behalf of the company to deviate in structure of alignment away from the formerly used prototypes most especially without official notice and authorization.

This kind of deviation from the former norms of the company structures might be regarded as false, misrepresentation, impersonation and forgery by the public even when it authentic. However, in the professional presentation of documented information, it is important to revisit

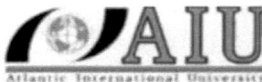
the templates and if there seem to be general changes then more binding attachments should be considered for acceptance.

3. Conciseness

It is a fact at a certain degree that the English language to the majority of the people around the world is a second language if not the third one. This implies that the language may not always be accurately grasped by the audience and possibly not well mastered by the writer most especially if he or she is not of English native (Blackwell, & Martin, 2011).

The aspect of conciseness has been attacked at a certain extents in the writing process by mistakes of exaggerated content, complicated phrases, excessive usage of jargons, misplaced tones, poor sentence linkage and essay transitions etc. it should be noted that excessive usage of jargons doesn't imply that the document text is of high profile. However, such texts instead makes comprehension and discourages the readers that continuously find the difficulty while looking for the hidden meanings. To attain a proficient conciseness in constructing a written professional text it is important to meet the following demands;

- Content overflow and control: - It is advisable in the professional paradigm to always limit the content of information presented on the written format. Perhaps the following examples can suffice this explanation;
- ➢ *Because of* = ~~based on the fact that~~
- ➢ ~~There were~~ *several subjects* ~~who~~ *completed...*
- ➢ ~~It should be noted that~~ = *nevertheless...*
- ➢ ~~In the event of~~ = *if*
- ➢ *Many* ~~different~~ *groups*
- ➢ ~~In close~~ *proximity... etc.*

In the example, outlines given above most of the common issues under discussion have been tackled for instance content reduction, reducing on over complicated phrases, elimination of the surplus words, active forms are favored more than the passive ones, and finally the application of linking words.

In addition to conciseness the written work is more credible when the grammatical principles, correct word spellings, vocabulary control usage are well followed as recommended according to the known norms. To achieve this aspect the modern digital and computerized word processing programs such as Microsoft office word (MS-Office word) can be employed to guide in spell check, grammatical corrections and conversion of passive to active phrases.

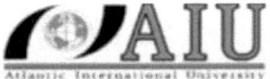

4.2 The APA recommended writing style

The American psychological association (APA) has invented writing guidelines over the years onto which standard manuscripts and text papers from electronic word processing can be produced in their best preciseness and admirable format. The APA style is not a limit line for professional and intellectual writing but rather a mean of standardization or calibration that serves to aid in producing excellent documented work both large, medium and small text papers.

The rules of the APA handbook cover different areas in most of the common types of text work i.e. concept papers, thesis papers, assignment papers, survey reports, publications, experimental reports and others. The guidelines and rules of the APA writing style cover areas such as:

- Paper layout (size, boundary margins, numbering patterns, page layout format etc)
- Text or character alignment (spacing, paragraphing, line spacing, title and header arrangement)
- Content of paper (preciseness, vocabulary, grammar, spellings, acronyms, abbreviations, essay flow and citations)
- Referencing (quotations, bibliography, and citations)
- Paper organization

The cardinal importance in this method of writing is that it encourages the usage of a single style that is known and recognised universally and for this reason it is easy for the reader to quickly point out the areas of interest and locate them while navigating the paper. The APA style is not limited to psychology studies but its importance can be extended in a variety of studies such as social sciences, nursing, business, administration, public relations etc.

It has been suggested by evidence that in the usage of the APA style it is easy to understand the different papers produced by various individuals even from different locations or institutions all over the world. What the APA style does is to ensure that all the written or electronic text manuscripts have a uniform character or features that will make easily graded if they study papers and possibly credited if they are more or less assignment for learners.

The main distinction that differentiates the APA writing style from other approaches is its ability to enhance creativity in the text works and emphasizing the writer to stick to the intellectual norms of writing. This means that the style helps to ground the learner or the student in intellectual development while designing or structuring sentences.

While writing according to the set rules which does not necessarily imply autocracy or directive in their format and adhering to them isn't harder and with consistence on these paradigms the individual writer becomes more acquainted until they no longer make life hard but instead they work for the benefit.

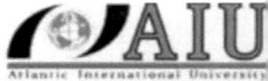
4.2.1 General formats of papers in the APA style

The different types of paper work demands for particular methods of approach since each may vary in requirement and structuring. The approach and organization of an experimental report paper is quite different from the techniques in designing an academic assignment text works. The challenges seem to be broad due to the difference in studies and requirements and unfortunately all these might not be discussed in this brief concept paper but instead for better comprehension of these technicalities the principal parts to be found in a professional writings are to be considered herein.

The APA Title page features and layout format

❖ The Title Page (layout and contents): This page for both experimental reports and the other professional work sheets should show the following features;

(a) The layout format should be A4 and side sentences starting 1inch away from the page boarder at each side.

(b) Title of the paper indicating the topic under discussion and the theoretical issues in the subtitle. The length of the Title used should be about 10-12 words long and centered in the middle of the page.

(c) The author's name and the institutional affiliation both capitalized. The institution of affiliation could be the college or organisation where the resulting work was achieved or carried out from. All these should be middle centered and below the title.

(d) A running head containing at least not more than 50 characters that are extracted from the topic title and this should be located in the top right corner of the page.

(e) The page number at the rear top right corner of the page

The importance of this format is that it presents the necessary details of the written work for the reader to easily identify the author, topic and organisation affiliations of the paper without difficulty. The deviations which are likely to be included by individuals might include underlining of the title, usage of figures (though these can be included in form of logos), unnecessarily long titles, and alignment of the details in a different order. All these deviations should be eliminated or if they are to retained it should be done under the directions of the academic advisor or any other person with such jurisdictions (Joyce, n.d.). . An example of the recommended title page required in the APA style can be observed from the figure below.

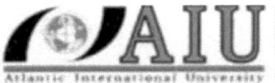
High Unemployment in Europe 1

Current Event Analysis

"High unemployment in Europe"

Edward Lambert

Atlantic International University

October 2013

Figure 6: Format of the standard APA style Title page

4.2.2 General contents of the literature review paper and the experimental report

These two types of official text works have considerable differences in requirements due to the post activities carried while building them. They represent the final findings or outcomes from the study activities to the reader for discretion and reference. In the common class literature review, the following contents are basic;

- The title page as shown in figure 7
- The general introductory section consisting of descriptions, explanations, and expository discussions
- The list of references for the citations, quotations, borrowed ideas and any other intellectual property of the second party

However, this arrangement should be used under the directions and guidelines of the instructing person. More information on such arrangements can also be found in the current APA tool kit for better formatting. On the other hand, the experimental report work is quite more broad and includes a variety of information such as below;

- The title page (see figure 7)

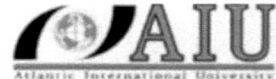
- An abstract
- Introduction
- Method
- Results
- The discussion of the study
- The list of references used in the study
- Figures and tables in mandatory in the study
- Appendix only where necessary

General contents and alignment of APA style fonts

❖ Headings:- These show the transition of titles and subtitles in the text paper at a hierarchy pattern depending on the levels contained. Common text papers have two levels where the first level is the heading 1 which is also bigger than heading 2 in the second level. Some bulky papers may extend up to three levels and in all these cases, each next heading has a smaller level in the index or the table of contents and throughout the essay.

❖ Fonts: - The APA writing style emphasizes the usage of a uniform type of font throughout the document and discourages the artistic applications of variable styles while typesetting professional text papers for official use. The universally recommended type of fonts for professional document presentation are; Arial and Times New Romans. In addition, these characters should be written with uniform size (12pt) though this may be altered while entering in the headings that may require large sizes but only for headings.

❖ Figures and Tables: - All the tables and figures should be properly labeled or titled as they descend for example table1, table 2 or in case of figures then figure 1, fig 2 etc. in proceeding contexts of the paper these should be referred to as indicated above (as shown in figure 1) and little details should be written or explained about their characteristics (American Psychological Association, 2009)

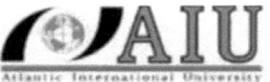
The information details in the different parts of the documents are also important in the professional writing style and hence requires special attention. The APA formatting style in official documents helps the writer to place the information where exactly it is supposed to be located. Take for example the following considerations;

❖ An abstract

This is a brief summary of the entire text paper written at the beginning of the work and should carry very little words (about 120 words). Repetitions of the title should be excluded there in order to minimize redundancy and spare space. However, in most papers the abstract is not mandatory therefore, in any case of its inclusion it is better to consider consultations from the instructor (American Psychological Association, 2009).

The information included in the abstract should be precise and brief showing only the necessary details that can catch the immediate attention of the reader since it is always used in the public display if in case it is for publication purposes. A mere class literature abstract should include information such as the problem under investigation and the general conclusion of your study, in case of the experimental report information may certainly include; problem under investigation, subjects of the investigation, methods used, findings obtained from this study and also the implications of the findings.

2. An introduction

This section varies depending on whether the paper is a literature or an experimental report paper and this there determines what type of information is to be included and how to arrange it. It is important to note that the introduction comes after the abstract and it contains the background information of the subject of the paper where it generally gives descriptions and explanations of the principal parts of the subject for both the experimental reports and common literature reviews .(American Psychological Association, 2009)

The size of the introduction vary also from whether it is a literature review or an experimental report (research work) and where more details are called for it is applicable to creating multiple headings in to subsection it for better comprehension by the reader.

In general terms it is important not to forget mentioning the importance of the study in the introduction as this creates more curiosity for the reader and describe the most important parts of the study only if in case it is an experimental report paper.

3. The Discussion Section

This acts as the expository section where most of the findings are handled or perhaps more explained. Assuming that the results have already been obtained and stipulated in the result

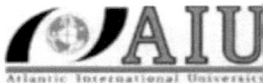
section and the methods used described already in the introduction an in the methodology section then the discussion takes the role of paraphrasing these issues for the reader.

Aspects like interpretation and evaluation of the findings are of great importance in the discussion section and these are used as parameters for addressing the questions or the problems raised during the experimental or study process. The APA style recommends the partitioning of the discussion into the following parts for conciseness and discrete work:

(a) Part 1: The review of the hypothesis and the results obtained. The hypothesis must have been mentioned in the methodology with all its features and the results are repeatedly overviewed in this section.
(b) Part 2: discussing the findings in relation to the literature context and at the same time addressing the limitations of the study
(c) Part 3: summarizing the contribution of the study to the literature and suggesting future trends of analysis.

4. The Recommendation

This is always a brief text pointing out some of the crucial matters from the study discussion and other sections of the document. The recommendation is important in reminding the reader the most important issues discussed and helps to suggest future proposals in helping to improve on the current outcomes (American Psychological Association, 2010).

The recommendations can also be used to identify the areas of weakness or the challenges associated in the methods, anomalies in the outcomes or deviations from the normal patterns and these should be used as the basis for suggesting better changes. (Check the recommendation at the end of this study for comparisons)

4.2.3 Dealing with Quotations, paraphrasing, summarizing and Citations
Quotations are phrases contributed by other individuals, which are then borrowed and applied in someone's work for better comprehension and exposition of the subject or topic under investigation or study. Any quotation borrowed from another person's findings should only be used as long as citations of the contributor or owner are to be included.

The APA style does not actually limit the size of the quotations to be used which on the other hand remains under the requirements of the paper and the guidelines stated by the instructor. However, constructing the paper where entirely 100% of it is quotations carries no meaning and for this reason there should be revised guidelines to prevent this anomaly.

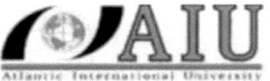
The citation of the quotations can be written after or before the quotation and this has no fixed approach though the citations should include the author and the date of the publication.

❖ **Paraphrasing** is the repetition of the author's words into someone's own words. Paraphrasing should only be used when the writer properly understands the author's concept. Consider the following remarks while paraphrasing;

- The key terms from the author's work should put in "quotes"
- Only select the portions appropriate in your explanations
- Prefer using your own style while discussing (Malmsfors et al. 2004)

❖ **A Summary** is a limited overview of what the author says in one's own words. In other words, it is a brief account from the author but digested in another process by the writer. Consider the remarks below in summarizing;

- it should always remain consistent with the original meaning of the author
- key terms from the author to used should be enclosed in quotations
- the original order of the context should followed

❖ **Quotations** represent borrowed words from another author and they should be arranged in the following way;
- quotation marks should be used in case words are extracted directly from the authors work ("quote")
- Quotation marks closing the quoted phrase should come before the parenthetical reference whereas the periodicals and commas come after the parenthetical reference ex. "quote" (Peter, 1998, p.5).
- However, characters such as question marks, exclamation marks that end the quote should be placed before the closing the quotation marks and hence the comma or a periodical in this case is required after the parenthetical reference.
- The block quotations (quotations with more than 40 words) are double spaced, indented on the left 0.5 inches and quotation marks are not to be included.

❖ **In-text reference citations** are written within the text work whenever the author's contributions are borrowed. The considerations below should be emphasized;
- Parenthetical references in the text work should include the author's surname and the year of publication ex. (Vonshens, 1976)
- When direct quotations are used then the page number should be included ex: (Vonshens, 1976, p.324)

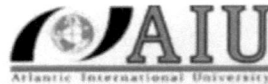
4.2.4 The APA Referencing Styles

Referencing in this criteria aims at indicating the source of the information cited in the text paper for the reader to easily and quickly locate or retrieve that information without difficulty. The process of referencing eliminates discrediting of the document due to plagiarism and improves on the authenticity of the work in the modern world.

Referencing should be presented at the end of the paper on a fresh page, page centered and with the capitalized title. The references cater for the citations and quotations inserted in the document essay as borrowed from other authors in other words all citations should be referenced at the end and all references in the list must be cited in the document text (Malmsfors et al. 2004).

Ethically, referencing protects the rights of ownership and serves to recognise the contributions of other individuals and hence mentioning their contributions without referring to their personality implies intellectual piracy and lack of authenticity. Most of the publications have been entered in the online databases with the details of their origin, author, title, date of their publication and the addresses hence the writer should not find difficulty in stating these features most especially if the work is electronic oriented. The most important information to be included in the reference list includes the following:

➢ The name(s) of the author(s) inverted and capitalized or the institution, organisation, group that created the work
➢ The date (year) during which the work was published
➢ The title of the work and sometimes the subtitle if provided
➢ The place where the work was published from
➢ The publisher of the work
➢ Information that aid the reader to retrieve the work more easily such as the URL, website, for web pages (American Psychological Association, 2009)

Nevertheless, it should be noted that works for referencing vary in type and this factor can alter the approach used while referencing for instance books, web pages, magazines, journals, videos, audios, eBooks, newspapers, etc. (Matthews, et al. 2000) .

Some of the basic rules to follow in referencing according to the APA writing style include;

i.   The authors name must be inverted (last names first) and all the names and initials must be given while capitalized.
ii.   The reference list should be arranged in alphabetical order regardless of the sections of citation
iii.   The author should always be mentioned first except if he or she is anonymous
iv.   Each reference should be entered on a new line while indented
v.   Titles should always be underlined or in italics

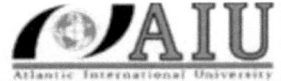
These rules however, vary with the type of work being referenced.

4.2.4 Examples of the APA Referencing Styles

Table 2: Showing Examples of the APA styles in referencing

Referencing a Book (non-periodical)												
Author	.	(year)	.	Book Title	.	Place of publication	:	Publisher			.	

Chapter or part of a Book												
Chapter Author	.	(year)	.	Chapter Title	.	In	Book editor(s) {Ed/Eds}	,	Book Title	(page range)	.	Place Of Publication	:	Publisher	.

Article in the periodical									
Author	.	(year)	.	Article title	.	Periodical title	,	Volume (issue)	,	Page range	.

Newspaper article								
Author	.	(year, month & day)	.	Article title	.	Newspaper name	,	Section and page(s)	.

Motion picture											
Producer name	.	Producer	, &	Director name	.	(Director)	.	(year)	.	Motion Picture Title	[Motion Picture]	.	Country of origin	:	Studio	.

Online article periodical with DOI (Digital Object Identifier)											
Author	.	(year)	.	Article Title	.	Periodical Title	,	Vol (issue)	,	Page Range	.	doi	:	XX.XXX

Periodical Online Article Without DOI									
Author	.	(year)	.	Article title	.	Periodical title	,	Volume(issue)	,	Page range	.	Retrieved from	URL

Article on website (no date)								
Author	.	(n.d.)	.	Article title	.	Retrieved from	Month day year	,	From	URL

Extracted From American Psychological Association. (2009)

Recommendations

As it would be postulated in any sector of intellectual practice that writing is a form of active communication involving the integration of various skills which in most cases are acquired then this ideology does not forego the need to consider irony in the discourse.

What sets a line of difference in the written communication while comparing the current norms with the ancient setting is that ancient times considered writing as a degree of great attention and awareness only undertaken during critical phenomenon and involving legendary skills.

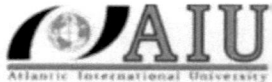
However, this fact has tremendously changed in the current pattern which has made writing to get involved in purposes of entertainment, awareness, statutory demarcations and other dimensions. Nevertheless it is these extensions that have posed a challenge of diverting the style: a factor which in so many cases could turn or arouse a stage of contention.

Important still, it should be noted that in the natural aspect of human communication to which also the writing avenue is attached the main factors that should be considered to choose or to assess the effectiveness of the method are audience and compatibility and in this case the former determines the later. Factually, while winning the attention of a particular community it is always vital to determine and analyse the type of audience involved and most especially the targeted group. The audience type can be distinguished or identified on parameters of age groups, gender orientations, educational levels or intellectualness, professional dimension or its relevancy to the topic under communication. The attentiveness of the audience also produces effective results aimed at in the process of communication and this attention can only be scored if the information is being conveyed to the targeted and exact audience.

Nevertheless, the type of the audience targeted and capturing it matters a lot in determining the compatibility of the written methods and guidelines followed therein. The public health sector mainly deals with public affairs and to be more precise and random the health aspect of the community which is considered as a fundamental aspect for human existence and this is what make such communication critical and of great importance. Due to the broadness of the public health paradigm involving a variety of technocrats, many anomalies and non-common trends of written information are likely to arise and these in most cases carry meaningful knowledge to the mass. However, this sort of technical writing is undigested and hence requiring more scientific techniques of interpretation which may not be occasionally or commonly dwell with the perception of the general public hence posing a need to further break it into simpler formats that are easily understandable by the targeted individuals (Booth, 1993) .

Consider for instance the raw facts that could result from an epidemiological research on disease or health prevalence in the community that if directly presented to the public in mere illustrations of data graphs and concept cover lines literally mean nothing. Consider also the possible outcomes that would result from the clinical trials on placebo drug developments carried in a random public research process. Such work commonly if not evenly produce terminologies and stoichiometric presentations that are rare not only to the illiterate but more so to the intellectuals from different professionals will not regarded as smart or accurate presentations but rather they face the challenge of being neglect since the uninformed parties will consider them irrelevant.

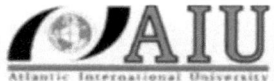

Conclusion

Fathoming still is the commonly unachievable trend that could be faced in the future developments and dynamics of the public health profession is the possible failure to communicate adequately to the targeted audience and this can get worse if the form of communication is under the written dimensions.

In spite of the simplicity that can result from consistent practice of a particular communication method either oral or written the fact remains both of these two dimensions have their limitations that can result into far reaching effects. For instance if in case comparison is made between these two modes of communications basing on the parameter of consistence, attentiveness and accountability then the written information preferably triumphs due to its possible positive features. The form of communication that promotes consistence and preciseness is not oral but rather written and if in case oral is preferred due to uncertain circumstances then extreme effort has to be applied to achieve the accuracy that can easily be achieved in the written format with less difficulty (Booth, 1993).

In a nutshell, the area of weakness associated with the writing paradigm result from its advantages still say for example consistency in which case if the message produced earlier requires alteration and editing for formality it may hardly be possible to reverse the already circulated material. However, this challenge also provides us with the possible solution which is to encourage adaptation to the recommended and global norms that are easily comprehended by the public (Matthews & Matthews, 2008).

Therefore, these global standards and recommendations in writing are the turning points which cause the need for revising the professional skills in scientific and intellectual writing that should be adapted for effective communication through the written format.

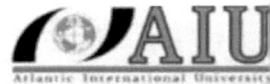

References

1. American Psychological Association. (2009). Mastering APA style: Instructor's resource guide (6th edition). Washington, DC: American Psychological Association.
2. American Medical Association Manual of Style (1998). A Guide for Authors and Editors, 9th ed.; Williams & Wilkins: Baltimore.
3. American Psychological Association. (2010). Publication manual of the American Psychological Association (6th edition). Washington, DC: American Psychological Association.
4. Blackwell, J. & Martin, J (2011). A Scientific Approach to Scientific Writing: illus. Springer
5. Booth V (1993). Communicating in science: writing a scientific paper and speaking at scientific meetings. Cambridge University Press, Cambridge, UK
6. Colomb, Gregory G., and Joseph M. Williams. (1985). Perceiving structure in professional prose: a multiply determined experience. In Writing in Non-Academic Settings, (eds). Lee Odell and Dixie Goswami. Guilford Press, pp. 87-128.
7. Eva Von Dassow .(n.d.). On Writing the History of Mesopotamia. Colorado: Colorado State University.
8. Gopen, George D. (1990). The Common Sense of Writing: Teaching Writing from the Reader's Perspective. To be published.
9. Gustavii B (2008). How To Write And Illustrate A Scientific Paper. Cambridge University Press, New York, NY
10. Joyce, A. S. (n.d.). Research letter: Canadian Group Psychotherapy Association. Retrieved October 26, 2009, from http://www.cgpa.ca/Research-Letter
11. Malmsfors B, Garnsworthy P, Grossman M (2004). Writing and presenting scientific papers. Nottingham University Press, Nottingham
12. Matthews JR, Matthews RW (2008). Successful scientific writing: a step-by-step guide for the biological and medical sciences. Cambridge University Press, New York, NY
13. Matthews, Janice R.; Bowen, John M.; Matthews, Robert W (2000). Successful Scientific Writing: a Step-by step Guide for Biomedical Scientists, 2nd ed; Cambridge University Press: New York.